Core Centered Care

*A 15-week devotional guide
exploring core character qualities for
health care professionals*

By Daniel Haifley, Th.D., D.D.

Table of Contents

Introduction..........*page 5*

I Corinthians 13..........*page 7*

And have not charity..........*page 9*

Charity suffereth long..........*page 13*

And is kind..........*page 19*

Envieth not..........*page 25*

Vaunteth not itself, is not puffed up..........*page 31*

Doth not behave itself unseemly..........*page 37*

Seeketh not her own..........*page 43*

Is not easily provoked..........*page 52*

Thinketh no evil........*page 58*

Rejoiceth not in iniquity..........*page 62*

Rejoiceth in truth........*page 66*

Beareth all things..........*Page 73*

Believeth all things..........*page 79*

Hopeth all things..........*page 85*

Endureth all things..........*page 89*

"Although the days are busy and the workload is always growing, there are still those special moments when someone says or does something, and you know you've made a difference in someone's life. That's why I became a nurse."

Diane McKenty

Introduction

Why did you start this journey of caring for other people? Was it the salary? Was it the long and strange hours? Or do you just have an internal desire to help people?

More than likely, if you are reading this, you, and all those like you, have arrived at this point from different backgrounds and circumstances. However, the common thread that joins you together is a desire, built into you by your Creator, to help people.

As a caregiver, there are times when your humanity envelopes you. You might be discouraged and ready to quit. This doesn't mean that you are a bad person, but what it does mean is that you need to take care of yourself. Regular maintenance spiritually and emotionally will help you stay the kind of person you were when you first entered this profession. And, hey– do you remember that excited, bright-eyed, young medical student who had all kinds of dreams and ambitions? Don't laugh at that person. That is the good part of who you are. That was when you were strong.

This lesson book is about making you strong again. It's about remembering who you are and who you want to be. It's about establishing your priorities and perspectives, and, yes, it is based on the Bible—particularly one chapter (I Corinthians 13) which sums up all of the Christian core values into one simple list.

The health care industry has realized the need to help nurses in personal areas beyond academic medicine. For example, The Massachusetts Department of Higher Education has developed a curriculum that is serving as a model to train the nurse of the future. A simple initialism, KAS, has been invented to define the three core competencies that nurses need to develop.

"K" stands for KNOWLEDGE. This is the part where you go to school and plow through lectures, text books, charts, and all the technical jargon necessary to declare you a nurse.

"A" stands for ATTITUDE. It has become abundantly clear that nursing is more than knowledge; it is also about conduct, outlook, interpersonal relationships, and self-worth.

"S" stands for SKILLS. Skills is an application of the knowledge and attitude. It is where the training becomes practice and where the textbook becomes the real world. It is where your daily work becomes measurable experience.

Sometimes, due to your knowledge and experience, you come face to face with circumstances that test your attitude to the core. Others in your shift or circle of caring become affected by the same stress that you are under, and gradually a toxic environment ensues.

When this happens, fall back to the tried and true principles of these lessons. Reconnect with your purpose and priorities, and find satisfaction, once again, in the thing that you do.

You must take care of yourself or you will quickly be unable to care for others.

-DH

"*Though I speak with the tongues of men and of angels, and have not charity, I am become as sounding brass, or a tinkling cymbal. And though I have the gift of prophecy, and understand all mysteries, and all knowledge; and though I have all faith, so that I could remove mountains, and have not charity, I am nothing. And though I bestow all my goods to feed the poor, and though I give my body to be burned, and have not charity, it profiteth me nothing.*

Charity suffereth long,
and is kind;
charity envieth not;
charity vaunteth not itself,
is not puffed up,
Doth not behave itself unseemly,
seeketh not her own,
is not easily provoked,
thinketh no evil;
Rejoiceth not in iniquity,
but rejoiceth in the truth;
Beareth all things,
believeth all things,
hopeth all things,
endureth all things.

Charity never faileth: but whether there be prophecies, they shall fail; whether there be tongues, they shall cease; whether there be knowledge, it shall vanish away. For we know in part, and we prophesy in part.
But when that which is perfect is come, then that which is in part shall be done away. When I was a child, I spake as a child, I understood as a child, I thought as a child: but when I became a man, I put away childish things.
For now we see through a glass, darkly; but then face to face: now I know in part; but then shall I know even as also I am known. And now abideth faith, hope, charity, these three; but the greatest of these is charity."
-I Corinthians 13-

"God gave burdens; he also gave shoulders."

Yiddish Proverb

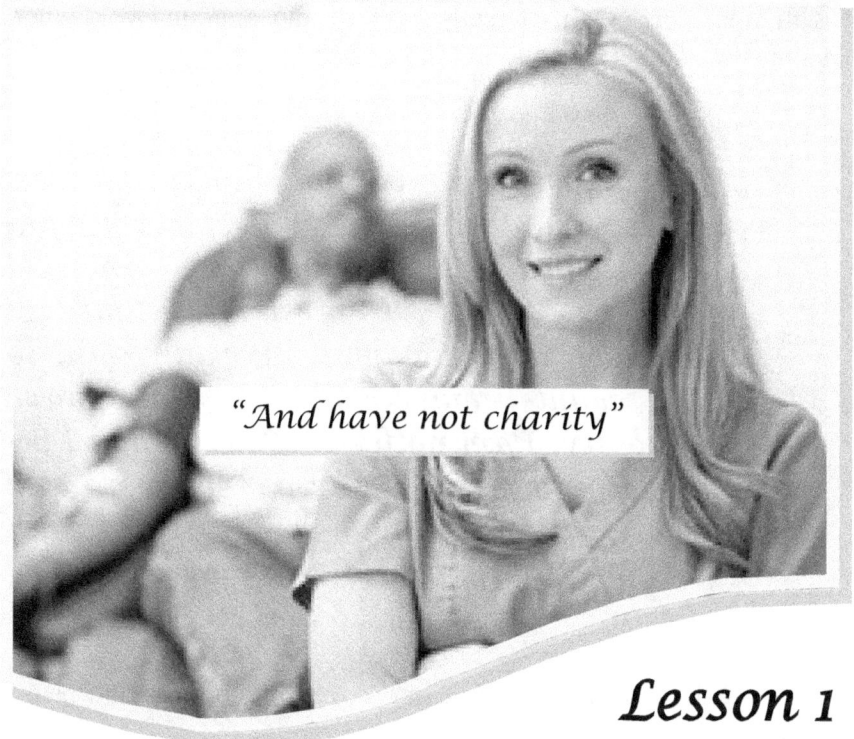

"*And have not charity*"

Lesson 1

What is Charity?

The original word in this chapter could be translated *love*. In fact, most translators use that word when translating this chapter. However, the word *charity* seems to cover a broader scope than the word *love*.

For example, if you were to give a homeless person something to eat, you would consider that to be *charity*, not *love*. However, that simple act of kindness is the love of God flowing through you to someone else. You are being used by God as the answer to someone's prayer. It is *love*, but you might not think of it as such.

Charity is the action intrinsically linked to the emotion. It is a good thing done from a good heart. According to the following verses, *charity*, is the core value of life. You will find satisfaction with your work, with yourself, and with those around you, when you make *charity* the cause of your effects.

*"Though I speak with the tongues of men and of angels, and have not charity, **I am become as sounding brass, or a tinkling cymbal.** And though I have the gift of prophecy, and understand all mysteries, and all knowledge; and though I have all faith, so that I could remove mountains, and have not charity, **I am nothing.** And though I bestow all my goods to feed the poor, and though I give my body to be burned, and have not charity, **it profiteth me nothing."*** I Cor. 13:1-3

Let's break down this passage into three simple parts and pause for some reflection on why we do what we do.

I. Without charity I am empty.

The first verse in I Corinthians 13 speaks of communication. If we can communicate well—even in more than one language— and don't have charity at our core, we are as wind in a brass instrument or the passing sound of a cymbal. Both are temporary noises that go away and are forgotten.

If the excitement has worn off, and you don't get the satisfaction that you once did, then maybe your focus is wrong.

II. Without charity I am nothing.

The next verse speaks of our vision for the future, our understanding and grasp of things around us, our knowledge and even our faith. These things all sound like a person that is well-rounded and someone you would want on your team. However, the writer goes on to say that without charity, none of this has any meaning.

Has your life lost its meaning? Has your position lost its mission-oriented feeling and become just a job?

III. *Without charity I receive no profit.*

The final statement in this section states that of every action I do—even to giving all I have to feed the poor and offering my life as a sacrifice—none of it will bring me any profit at all, unless it is motivated by the core value—charity.

> One person caring about another one, represents life's greatest value.
> **Jim Rohn**

Have you become cynical and hard to get along with? Have people become a bother to you? Then you are no longer profiting from the thing you are doing.

Reflection
What am I going to do to regain my Core balance?

For myself

For my co-workers

For my patients

"Compassion automatically invites you to relate with people because you no longer regard people as a drain on your energy."

Chogyam Trungpa

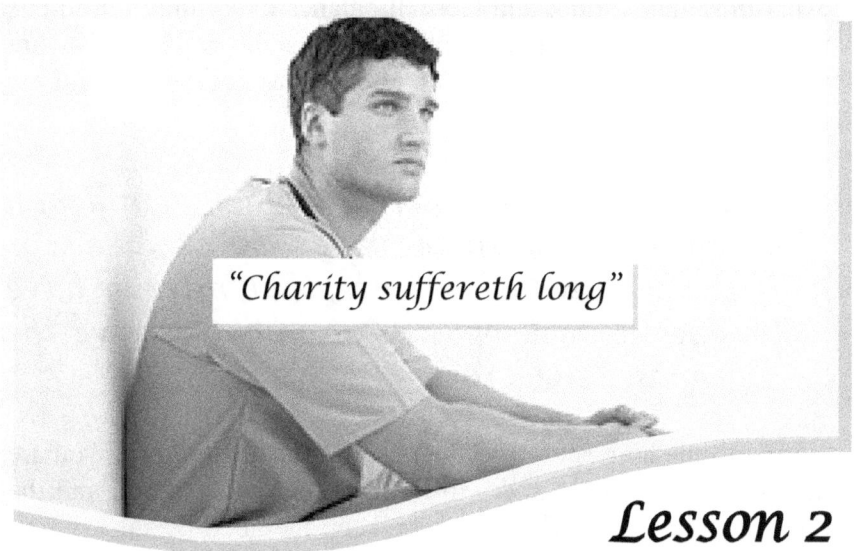

"*Charity suffereth long*"

Lesson 2

We live in a culture that thrives on instant gratification. We fuss and fume if our fast food is not quite fast enough. We get upset if the check-out lanes are too long. We're even irritated if the internet, which provides instant answers to our questions, delays a few seconds longer than we think it should.

However, the caregiving profession does not produce instant results. It does not receive instant feedback. The results sometimes are not even visible and might even be non-existent.

Patience, then, is something that must be developed if you are planning on staying in this profession for any length of time. It does not come naturally, and usually comes painfully, but it can be acquired by determination. Let me say, also, that it will make the difference between a top-notch caregiver and a mediocre one.

I. Patience will give you what you want after you have done what you should.

Sometimes doing right can be frustrating. It may appear that the people that cut corners and try to gain favor in the wrong way are getting all of the benefits, but don't forget that God is watching everything that we do, and He will balance everything out in His time. He is the one that ultimately gives the rewards that are worth waiting for. The apostle in his letter to the Hebrews makes this point:

> *"Cast not away therefore your confidence, which hath great recompense of reward. For ye have need of patience, that, after ye have done the will of God, ye might receive the promise." Heb. 10:35-36*

Your attitude hinges on the understanding that everything you are doing is worth doing, and will be beneficial both to you and the one you care for. Maybe, you have been the good person who always does what is expected and never takes short cuts, yet you see nothing positive come from it. Don't throw away the confidence that you are a good caregiver. Don't get discouraged and say, "What's the use." Stay at it. You will receive your reward for doing right, even if it is not in this life.

II. Patience allows everything to develop perfectly in its proper time frame.

James tells us in his letter to let patience have her perfect work.

> *But let patience have her perfect work, that ye may be perfect and entire, wanting nothing. Jas. 1:4*

You can't force an apple to grow on a tree. It just happens when the tree is properly cared for. Giving it plenty of water, trimming the branches, and spraying it for insects will give the tree a chance to bear good apples, but still you must let it do its thing. You cannot will it to bear peaches if it is an apple tree, but you can help it to bear the best apples possible. You cannot force people to change. They are what they are. However, by investing in each person's life, and then allowing that investment to work, you will discover that you can help them be the best they can be.

If a circumstance seems to be careening out of control, invest the time and resources that you have available, and then allow that investment to work. You may not get out of the situation immediately, but you will find a way through it.

III. Patience requires waiting and accepts the circumstances as they are.

Life is 10% what happens to me and 90% how I react to it. **Charles Swindoll**

It might be easy to be patient on a short-term basis, but it is after a long–term case, when we have our breakdown. Remember what charity does? It suffers LONG.

Your expectation is usually what influences your stamina. If you have determined that it is a long-term investment, you can deal with it. If you plan on instant returns, and it becomes long-term, than you get discouraged. Let's just forget the short-term expectation for now and look at three different kinds of LONG-term patience.

A. "Be patient therefore, brethren, unto the coming of the Lord. Behold, the husbandman waiteth for the precious fruit of the earth, and hath long patience for it, until he receive the early and latter rain." Jas. 5:7

A husbandman is a farmer. He plants his crops, and then waits an entire season for the fruit of his labors. Maybe he goes out and waters the plants. Maybe he fertilizes. The whole time he is waiting, he is caring for what he has planted, but he is never expecting to receive a benefit until the end of the season. Caregiving in a hospital is very similar to it.

Someone is sick, and he is admitted for a short time. He is cared for, medicated for a season, and hopefully manifests a turn-around physically and then released. This could possibly be compared to a normal day in the life of a nurse.

B. *"Behold, we count them happy which endure. Ye have heard of **the patience of Job**, and have seen the end of the Lord; that the Lord is very pitiful, and of tender mercy." Jas. 5:11*

The story of Job is one of the most intriguing stories in all of history. He was a man that was very devout, and hated anything that was evil. He prayed and sacrificed for his children on a daily basis. Things suddenly started going wrong for him, and he had no idea why. Most of the story tells us of his struggle to understand why things had happened the way they had.

Job lost all of his wealth. His children were all killed in one accident. His wife even told him his faith was worthless and that he might as well curse God and die. We know there was a lesson being taught to Satan, but Job had no idea about the conversation that was going on in another realm. Yet, in all that happened to him, he never once spoke against God. He accepted his circumstances as if he deserved them, and in the end, God blessed him with twice as much as he had before the whole crisis took place.

Sometimes we can feel like we are getting too loaded down with all that is piled upon us. The proverbial "straw that broke the camel's back" has just been placed on our already-too-heavy burden. Just remember that the story is not finished yet. Get a grip on yourself, and trust the Lord with the future. You can live through the situation. There is an end to every storm.

C. *"Take, my brethren, **the prophets**, who have spoken in the name of the Lord, for an example of suffering affliction, and of patience."*
Jas. 5:10

The third kind of long-term patience is the kind that produces re-sults in the next generation. The problem is, it never produces re-sults that you can see in your lifetime. It might even produce re-sults which will never bring recognition to you—you will never be able to claim them on your resume, and you will never realize a bonus from them.

The prophets of the Old Testament are the ones from whom we draw inspiration here. They were men investing in something that would have universal implications that would not be realized or understood until long after they were dead. They would never see the results or even understand them. Some of them were literally killed for their message, and many were subjected to torture and deprivation. They might have even questioned God on occasion, but they still did what they were supposed to do when they were supposed to do it, and we are the beneficiaries of their faithful-ness.

Reflection
How can I let patience work?

In a short term situation
In something that is piling up
For future generations

"Caregiving often calls us to lean into love we didn't know possible."

Tia Walker

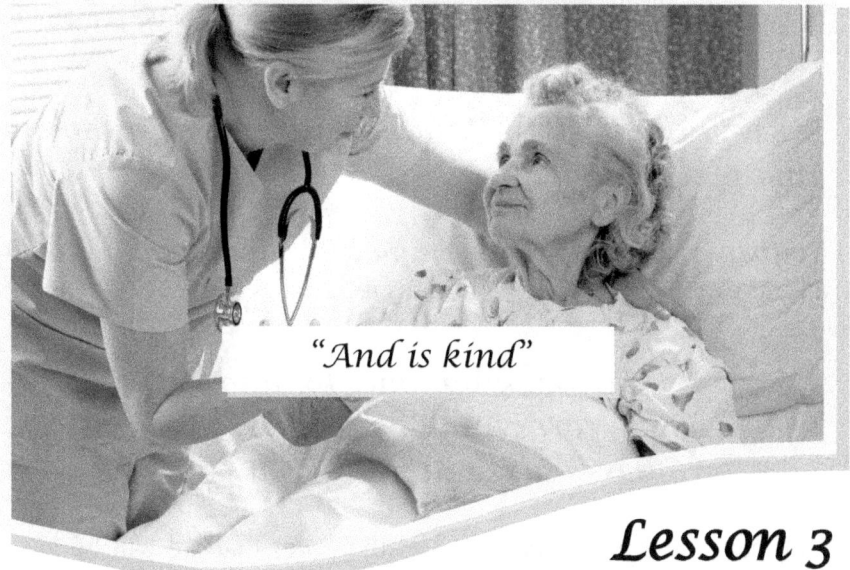

"*And is kind*"

Lesson 3

In 1993, Denver, Colorado experienced a summer filled with violence. Dozens of people were killed in gang-related shootings that included folks that were not involved in gangs at all. One victim was only 10 months old. As a response to this horrific season, an organization was formed called "The Random Acts of Kindness Foundation." (RAKF)

This foundation has grown way beyond a single community to include over 23 different countries. Schools are beginning to teach kindness on purpose. Research is being done on the long-term affects of kindness on people individually and on society overall.

What researchers have discovered is something that the Bible had already suggested a couple thousand years ago—that kindness is core to happiness, both to ourselves and to those with whom we interact.

It doesn't matter what your personality traits are, you can be a kind person. Researchers have discovered that kindness is a learned behavior. Maybe that is why the Bible gives us a command to be kind.

19

In the following outline we are going to explore some principles from the Bible that can help you become a kind person.

I. Being thankful for kindness to you will promote kindness from you.

You will be kinder when you realize that you have been treated in a kind way by others. In Ephesians 4:32 we read:

> *"And be ye kind one to another, tender-hearted, forgiving one another, even as God for Christ's sake hath forgiven you."*

You see, the Apostle Paul makes the point that we can be kind and forgive others because Christ has already forgiven us. Christ has been kind to us, and we are to use that as a motivation to be kind to others.

Lets talk about the kindness that has been shown to you.

> *"Let this mind be in you, which was also in Christ Jesus: Who, being in the form of God, thought it not robbery to be equal with God: But made himself of no reputation, and took upon him the form of a servant, and was made in the likeness of men: And being found in fashion as a man, he humbled himself, and became obedient unto death, even the death of the cross." Philippians 2:5-8*

How much has Jesus done for you? His kindness caused Him to lay aside the glory of heaven and to take on Himself the form of man. Why?... Just so that He could die to pay for your sins and mine. Not only has He forgiven our sin debt, but He has also guaranteed us a place with Him forever—a place where there is no more sorrow, nor crying, nor pain of any kind. Did He do this because we deserved it? No. He did it out of kindness.

"That in the ages to come he might shew the exceeding riches of his grace in his kindness toward us through Christ Jesus."

Ephesians 2:7

In another place, Paul challenges a friend to forgive his servant, and then adds,

"...albeit I do not say to thee how thou owest unto me even thine own self besides."

Philemon 19

Remembering the kindness that has been shown to you by someone else will, in turn, motivate you to be kind to others. By the way, thankfulness for the kindness shown to you, is not a natural feeling. It is a learned behavior. Stop and take notice what other folks have done for you. (*"Count your blessings name them one by one, and it will surprise you what the Lord has done."*)

II. Kindness from you produces more kindness in others.

We need to be aware that every act of kindness we do has a ripple effect. When we are kind to someone, that person is motivated to be kind to someone else. "Pay it forward," has become a common phrase which is simply about giving to someone who will in turn give to someone else.

We are creatures that thrive on imitation. We learn our behavior—even our speech patterns—by imitating other people. Kind behavior is learned in exactly the same way. As we are kind to others, we increase the potential for kindness in all those who watch us, and then our behavior becomes a model for them. Maybe kindness is a gift that you give; maybe it is a simple smile;

possibly it is just a pause in your busy schedule to recognize the needs and desires of another person. Kindness is not expensive. It is something that anyone can do, yet the results of it are far reaching.

Erin Brockovich became a household name after the 2000 feature film about her life was released. She is an environmental activist who spearheaded a massive law suit against a gas company for polluting the water in her home town of Hinkley, California. The gas company had to pay three hundred thirty-three million dollars to more than six hundred Hinkley residents who had been affected by its negligence.

There is another story about her that isn't so well-known. Erin had a teacher in school who discovered that she was dyslexic. Up to that point, she had failed in all of her classes. Her test papers were always F's. One day a teacher, named Kathy Borsa, called her up to her desk after a particularly disturbing failure. She took the exam paper and ripped it up, telling Erin that she had noticed she just learned differently then the other students. She then said, "Let me ask you these questions in a different way." She gave Erin the questions orally, and when she had discovered that Erin knew all of the answers, the teacher gave her an A+. According to Erin Brokovich, that day changed her life. She said that the kindness of that one teacher gave her the self-esteem to become the woman she is, and of course, the rest is history. What an influence you can have on the world by just a small act of kindness to one person!

III. *Kindness from you is expected by God.*

Jesus tells a story in Luke 17, about a servant who does exactly what he is supposed to do. The master comes in from the field after a hard day's work, and the servant provides him a seat and his supper. Then Jesus goes on to tell the disciples that most likely this servant would not even get a thank you from his master, because he was hired to do those things—those things were his duty. Then He continues with:

"So likewise ye, when ye shall have done all those things which are commanded you, say, We are unprofitable servants: we have done that which was our duty to do."

This story is vital to this lesson since it was not a random parable. Jesus had a purpose for saying this at that time. You see, He had just been telling the disciples what to do if someone wronged them. He said that if your brother sins against you and repents, you should forgive him. If he sins seven times in a day, and each time turns back to you for repentance, you should forgive him. Later Peter came to ask Him if seven times was the limit, and Jesus told him he should forgive seven times seventy times. That was a figure of speech which means that there is no limit to how many times you should forgive. The disciples responded with incredulity, "Increase our faith." Then Jesus told them this story. I understand from this that forgiveness is not an option for us. We don't get to choose if or not we forgive. It is our duty. In case He wasn't clear enough, He states at the end of the Lord's Prayer:

"But if you forgive not men their trespasses, neither will your Father forgive your trespasses." Matthew 6:15

Reflection

Who can I show kindness too?
Who do I need to forgive?

*"Forgiveness is not an occasional act:
it is an attitude."*

Martin Luther King Jr.

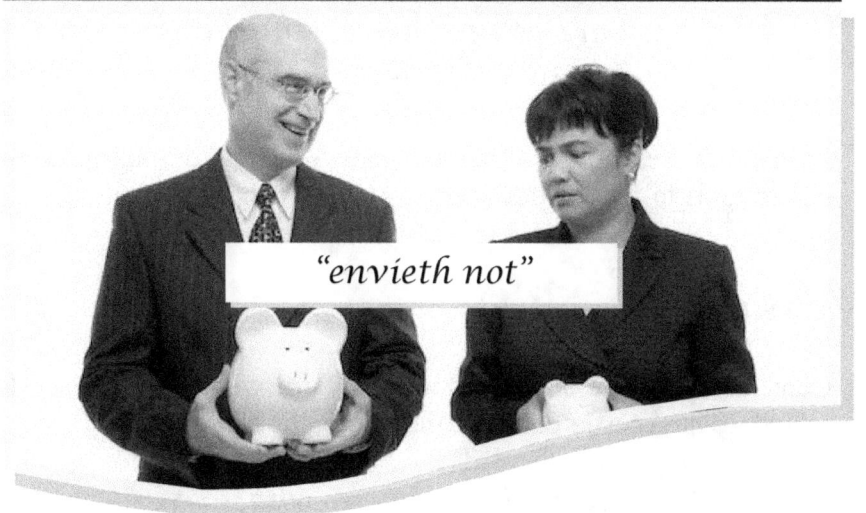

"envieth not"

Lesson 4

How do you feel when someone is promoted over you? How about if you know that this same person is not as qualified as you are to run the program? What if it is a supervisor that gets a special award for something **you** did? Do you like how those things make you feel?

King Solomon wrote down this statement in his list of proverbs,

> *"Wrath is cruel, and anger is outrageous, but who is able to stand before envy?" Prov. 27:4*

Envy will destroy everyone that is in its vicinity. If you are envious, it will destroy you. It will affect those who are closest to you. Oh, and if someone is envious of you, what can you really do about it?

Truthfully we all have an inclination to be jealous of someone else. God addressed this problem in the ten commandments:

*"Thou shalt not covet anything
that is thy neighbor's."*

In the New Testament, James explains to us that our spirit has a natural pull to be envious (James 4:5). So what do we do about this?

I. Learn to be content.

Contentment is not something we are born with. It is a learned attitude. The Apostle Paul told the Philippian church,

> *"...For I have learned, in whatsoever state I am, therewith to be content." Phil. 4:11*

A large dose of reality, thankfulness and trust in God, will help you down the road towards contentment.

Reality check—he who dies with the most toys still dies. Why are we always reaching for bigger and better? Usually we are motivated by those around us. We tell ourselves that we just want to fit in, but maybe, in reality, we are just giving in to envy.

Henry David Thoreau in his book, Walden Pond, wrote about an experiment he tried. He decided to see just how little money was really necessary to live. So he moved out away from society and set up a little shack by this particular pond. By the end of his experiment, he had made several conclusions. He discovered that every time someone else would get a raise, he would immediately raise his own standard of living, so that he never had quite enough to live on. If he were to become content with his current standard of living, and save the remaining money, he would eventually become quite wealthy. Contentment is a great benefit financially.

Do you know that godliness with contentment is great gain? Read what Paul told young Timothy along these lines: (I Tim. 6:6-9)

"But godliness with contentment is great gain. For we brought nothing into this world, and it is certain we can carry nothing out. And having food and raiment let us be therewith content. But they that will be rich fall into temptation and a snare, and into many foolish and hurtful lusts, which drown men in destruction and perdition."

If you could learn to be content with the food and clothes that are necessary for your life, you will find that everything else is just an added blessing. Your perspective on life will get straightened out, and you will find that you are not so prone to be envious of what someone else has.

II. Accept your own personal value.

The Bible (I Cor. 12:4-7) tells us that there are different kinds of gifts, different kinds of administrations, and different kinds of operations. In other words, everybody is different and has a different role to play. Each role that is played, is vital to the entire scheme of life. Each role can only be played by the individual to whom it belongs. If that individual is constantly looking at someone else's life, accomplishments, or reward, he will never realize his own potential.

One of our best cures for envy is acceptance of who we are and a focus on what we can do with what we have. If we spend our time developing ourselves and focusing on our uniqueness—even capitalizing on it—we will avoid the deep valley of envy. And, of course, we must not forget the value that God places on our lives.

- What is man that thou are mindful of Him?
- He sees the sparrow fall and we are valued more highly.
- The very hairs of our head are numbered.
- He knew all our parts before they were fashioned.

- Every breath is ordered by the Lord.
- His thoughts toward us are more than can be numbered.
- "For God so loved the world that He gave His only begotten Son, that whosoever believeth in Him, should not perish, but have everlasting life."

There is more. All of those things are stated in the pages of the Bible. Think how much God loves you! Even if you are not following Him the way you should, He is following every detail of your life. There is no reason for you to envy anyone else.

III. Realize that your efforts will produce results.

One of my favorite verses in the Bible is Galatians 6:9. It is a promise to those who will just put forth a little effort. Here is what it says:

> *"And let us not be weary in well doing: for in due season we shall reap, if we faint not."*

Sometimes it may seem that all of your hard work goes unnoticed. You see others being promoted around you or awarded things you don't think they deserve...but just remember, there is a righteous Judge who is watching all things. He is not a respecter of persons, but He is fair in all of His dealings. He has promised that He will reward you for the good you do, whether it be in this life or the next. Jesus said that if you would do something as small as give a cup of cold water in His name, or in the name of a disciple, you would receive a reward. Sowing seeds of discord, rebellion, bad attitudes, etc. will bring in a crop of negativity. A simple law of life is that you will reap from what you have planted. If you sow good things, you will reap good things. If you sow bad things, you will reap bad things.

The book of Psalms is the Jewish song book. King David is credited for writing most of the Psalms, but some of them he collected and added to his writings. One of those is Psalm 90, which was actually written by Moses. This chapter is a beautiful work of praise to God, but I'd like to draw your attention to the very last verse of the Psalm. After Moses has praised God for everything He has done in the creation, he says this as a prayer:

"And let the beauty of the Lord our God be upon us: and establish thou the work of our hands upon us; yea, the work of our hands establish thou it."

Moses is not asking God to miraculously bless his life. He is not asking for protection, neither for fame nor for fortune. Instead, he is pleading with the Almighty to look at the work of his hands. He is saying, "I am going to work hard, but I need you to bless my work like you have blessed your work." What a great plan for success! Work like it all depends on you; trust like it all depends on God. If you focus more on your efforts, trusting God to bring results, you will be able to enjoy the promotions that come to other people as well.

"Rejoice with them that do rejoice, and weep with them that weep." Romans 12:15

Reflection   *What has God given to me?*

Personal Blessings:
Personal Strengths:

"*A man's pride shall bring him low: but honour shall uphold the humble in spirit.*"

King Solomon

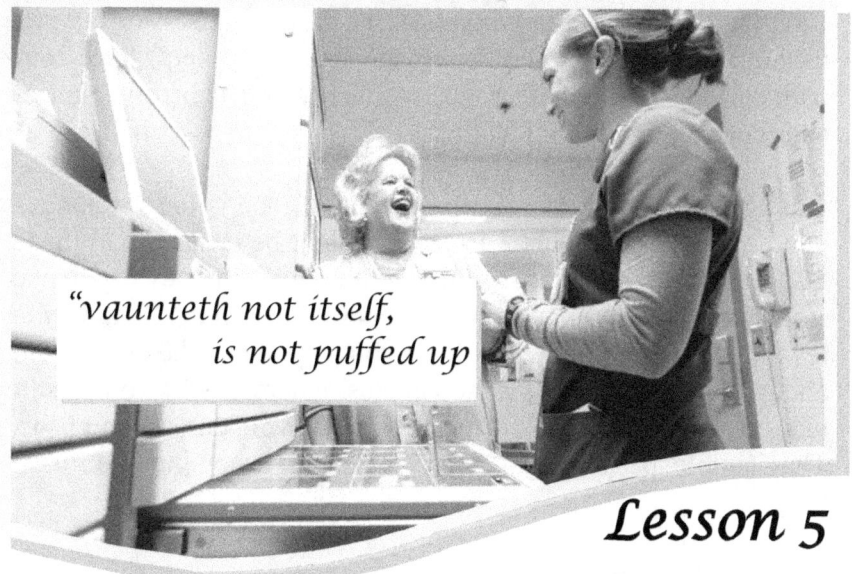

*"vaunteth not itself,
is not puffed up*

Lesson 5

"Vaunteth" is an old English word that simply means bragging. So then, one who is full of charity, this needful core value, is one who will not spend anytime bragging. Of course, the word, "vaunteth," has a little heavier meaning than "bragging." The exact definition is: "...a vain display of what one is, extravagant self -praise, show off. And vain means: "...having no real substance." It is not wrong for you to know what you can do, and it is not wrong to let others know what you can do—particularly in the environment you work in. But this "vaunting thing" is putting yourself on display for no other reason than to make people think highly of you. It is that moment when you want people to think you are really experienced or that you are really one of the greatest!

I'm sure you know someone who likes to turn every conversation to himself. Every story you tell, he has a counter story that's bigger and more exciting. He may think that he is a conversationalist, but, in reality, you think he is a bore. As a caregiver, this is a dangerous practice to be engaged in.

I have heard and known of several Critical Incident Stress Teams that have been called in to debrief first responders and multi-level caregivers. Later, those who sat in the debriefing sessions (which usually have been proven to provide significant help) have complained that the specialists just wanted to tell their own stories, and they weren't helpful at all.

Giving facts about your abilities or experience is fine, as long as you don't embellish them. In fact, it might be necessary at times. The team that you work with needs to know what they can expect from you. Those under your care also might need to know what level of care they can expect from you. If you feel the need to talk about yourself in this way, stop and ask yourself why you need to talk about yourself. Ask yourself, "What will this accomplish?" That simple pause might keep you from becoming the "party bore."

I. It is the original sin.

Before God created man, He created angels. According to the scriptures, Lucifer was the crowning creation. He was the most beautiful and talented of the angels. When he realized that he was greater than the others, he began to think of himself as if he were God. Notice how the prophet Isaiah described this moment.

> *"How art thou fallen from heaven, O Lucifer, son of the morning! how art thou cut down to the ground, which didst weaken the nations! For thou hast said in thine heart, I will ascend into heaven, I will exalt my throne above the stars of God: I will sit also upon the mount of the congregation, in the sides of the north: I will ascend above the heights of the clouds; I will be like the most High." Isaiah 14:12-14*

When Lucifer began to think of himself more highly than he ought to, he began to vaunt himself above all the other created beings. This led to his eventual downfall.

In the New Testament we are challenged not to think more highly of ourselves than we ought. A novice is not supposed to be put in a high position lest pride gets in his way, and he fall into "the condemnation of the Devil." The scripture warns us, time and time again, to be careful in this area, because it is dangerous ground.

II. It is the underlying reason for man's disconnect with his Creator.

Did you know that every culture has its altar? If you were to go to the darkest, most forgotten places in this world, you would find an altar of some kind (with sacrifices-peculiar to that area) built to a particular god of their choice.

The Bible says in Romans chapter one, that every creature understands the wrath of God. We are all born with this understanding. It is not something that we have to be taught; we just understand it. That's why there is an altar in every culture. Everyone knows we all are in trouble with someone somewhere because of the things we have done—those things that we hope no one ever finds out about. Religions have been formed in every culture to treat this problem. All of them have designed some way to make us feel better about ourselves by making sacrifices of some sort or another. People will make expensive trips to exotic places to find some connection with inner peace. Some folks will do degrading and painful things to themselves to demonstrate their desire to rid themselves of the terrible weight of guilt.

Paul goes on to explain in this chapter that the problem began when we knew God but didn't put Him in His rightful place. We became vain in our imaginations and started worshipping ourselves. After a time, God gave us over to our imaginations and let us try to depend on ourselves. As time has progressed man has gotten more and more vile, completely changing our nature and manipulating our purpose for our own good.

There is a cure. God said if we would humble ourselves, and pray, and seek His face, and turn from our wicked ways, then He would hear from heaven and would forgive our sins and heal our land.

Don't try to appear to be humble when you are not. That doesn't fix the problem. Genuinely humble yourself. Recognize what you are and what you are not. See the opportunities that you have been given as direct blessings from God. See your talents as gifts that you have been given to benefit others. This will change your perspective about yourself and will make you a better caregiver.

III. Focus on the Future.

Another thing that will help you with this problem would be to not spend so much time patting yourself on the back for previous accomplishments. While you should feel good about the positive things you have done, try to keep some of that just between you and God.

Here are a couple of verses that illustrate this point:

> *"Brethren, I count not myself to have appre-hended: but this one thing I do, forgetting those things which are behind, and reaching forth unto those things which are before, I press toward the mark for the prize of the high calling of God in Christ Jesus."*
>
> *Philippians 3:13 -14*

Here, Paul is telling us that the secret of his success is that he doesn't consider himself to be the expert. He doesn't think that he has arrived. Instead, he puts his accomplishments and failures behind him and doesn't dwell on them. He then puts all of his effort into the future, pressing towards the prize that God has promised to him. The word "press" that he uses in these verses is an old nautical term. Some of the old sailing ships relied completely on wind power to move. Sometimes a ship might get off course a little and lose the wind that was so essential and just drift for days. If a slight wind would come up, the captain would order a "press of sails." That meant that every available piece of cloth on the ship was to be used to catch the wind.

The idea that Paul is communicating here is that we should not put all of our energy into self promotion, but rather, raise every ability and resource to the wind of God's will, focusing on reaching the real prize—hearing God say, "Well done."

Reflection

How can I humble myself?
What kind of things can I do to make me a better caregiver?
What God given abilities do I have?

*"Some days there won't be a song in your heart.
Sing anyway."*

Emory Austin

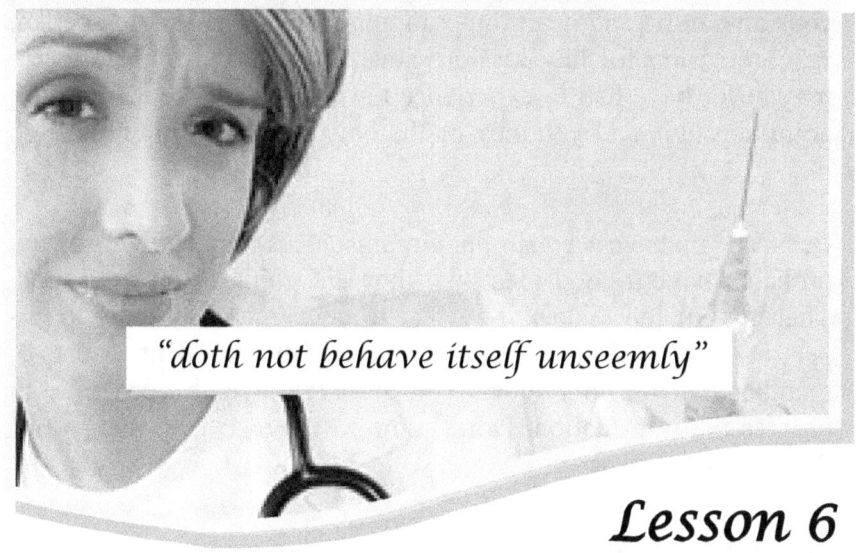

"doth not behave itself unseemly"

Lesson 6

Everyone has good days and bad days, but, as a healthcare professional, you do not have the privilege of being transparent with your feelings. You must, at all times, conduct yourself in a manner which brings reassurance and comfort to everyone around you. Some people may be difficult to deal with. Some may have a completely different world view than you, and some might even disgust you. You cannot let this affect your care of them. Your job is to give equal care and comfort to all, regardless of race, religion, age, health condition, sex, or any number of other factors.

The interaction between caregiver and patient is often referred to as "bed-side manner." This is the subject we will be dealing with in this lesson.

I. The Danger of Callousness

Over time, you develop coping mechanisms for the trauma that you experience. Sometimes the only way to deal with what you see on a daily basis. is to develop a clinical attitude towards everything. You stop seeing the pain and start looking at just the science of the situation. That may be the way you deal with it in your own mind and heart, but you must remember that the person you are caring for has possibly never been this road before. He may never have had to experience the trauma that he is currently going through, and you may be the only one to help him through it.

Because you have seen similar circumstances play out before, you probably have a good idea how they are going to turn out now. That is your job. You know what to do. You know what to expect. You know how the family is going to react. But... just remember that the individuals you are dealing with need time to process the information. Don't jump to the end; help them work through the process.

II. Bedside Manner

If you can succeed in making the patient feel comfortable and taken care of, you can sometimes speed up the recovery time. There are several elements that make up good "Bedside manner."

- Vocal tones This involves the pitch of your voice—the softness or harshness of it. The tone of your voice can affect the way you are perceived. It is something that can be practiced. There are many free internet lessons on developing good quality tones in your speaking voice. Be gentle.
- Body language Impatience can be communicated by your body language. Before you enter the room, disconnect from what just happened in the previous room. If you are upset at a co-worker or a family member, you can easily project this on to your next patient. First, give a greeting and introduction to every one in the room. Listen to them with your eyes. Look right at them while they are talking to you. Show a specific interest in their concerns. Make their visitors feel comfortable by making sure that they have a place to sit.
- Openness Don't act like you are trying to conceal anything. Give them all of the information that you can within the boundaries of your responsibility. Assure them that if you can't answer their questions you will find someone who can.

Most people are able to handle the details of a trauma, but they will soon get frustrated if they feel that you are holding back information.

- Presence Communicate the message that you are available for their every need. If you are tied up with an emergency in the next room, be sure to apologize for the inconvenience to the waiting patient. Assure them that it's ok to use the call button for anything at anytime. Ask the visitors in the room if you can get them coffee or water or anything. Sometimes providing little comforts makes all the difference in how the care is perceived.

- Time can be an illusion. If the doctor lets you know that he will be in to see the patient in one hour, leave room for error. If you tell them to expect him within two hours and twenty minutes, they will occasionally look at their clocks, but will try to understand that the doctor is busy and will get there soon. If he shows up in one hour, they will be immediately surprised and blessed that the time was less than expected, and they will feel like you can be trusted to put their interests as a high priority. But on the other hand, if you make promises that he will be here in one hour, and he is five minutes late, they will be frustrated.

III. Death Notifications

Don't forget that you have an excellent resource to help with death notifications. Many of your chaplains are trained specifically in this area and have had experience with this on numerous occasions. In the event that it falls to you to be involved in this difficult task here are some tips to remember:

- Make sure everyone is sitting down. An extreme blow to the emotions can sometimes cause a person to collapse and injure himself. When everyone is sitting down then tell them.
- Make sure you have the right family. Ask how each person is connected to the particular individual in question.
- Tell them what happened as best you can in layman's terms. Make sure that you are clear that the patient has died, but an-

nounce it in as gentle a way as you can.

- Refrain from using the "God card." Often well-meaning people try to explain away things that we don't understand by saying foolish things as: "God needed them more than you did." "It was their time to go." etc. Recognize that losing a loved one sometimes has no good explanation, and just doesn't make any sense at all.

- Don't tell them you understand, and don't tell them your personal stories. They feel like no one can understand their pain right at this moment. Tell them you are sorry for their loss, and then let them know you are there for them. Sometimes, they just need a shoulder to cry on.

IV. Life support issues

A living will helps the healthcare professional immensely when there is a question about life support. Don't be quick to "pull the plug." You have seen it before. You know that the family is draining their strength and emotions by just waiting by the bedside. You know that the end is inevitable. However, the family and friends need to go through the grieving process.

Usually when someone dies in the hospital, the family has an attachment to that room. It has become a security for them, and they feel like they are hanging on to their loved one just a little longer by staying in there. They feel like as soon as they leave the room all hope is gone, and so they will linger.

But all you think of is that **you** have a job to do. Maybe you need to get the room ready for the next patient. For you this job is completed and so can you move to the next task. Be careful, however, to remember your responsibility as a healthcare professional, to care for the needs of those who have been left behind. Call for a chaplain who can help the family move on to the next step, and who can guide them graciously to another place to collect themselves. During that time stay with them. Don't disconnect from the family too soon.

V. Donating body parts

This is a very difficult and sensitive area, and should only be handled by those qualified to discuss it. Never pressure someone to make a decision to donate the body parts of a loved one. If there is a living will, the decisions have already been made. You may have some time-sensitive decisions to make, but that is your job. Their job is to grieve. You want to save the next person, but the gift of organs is a noble thing that must be treated with much dignity.

Reflection

How long have I served as a care provider?
Have I gotten calloused to the pain I see every day?
How can I disconnect from situations in other rooms?
What should I do first when I enter a patient's room?
What do I do if I don't have an answer to their questions?
Whom should I call to help with spiritual and emotional needs?

"Compassion brings us to a stop,
and for a moment we rise above ourselves."

Mason Cooley

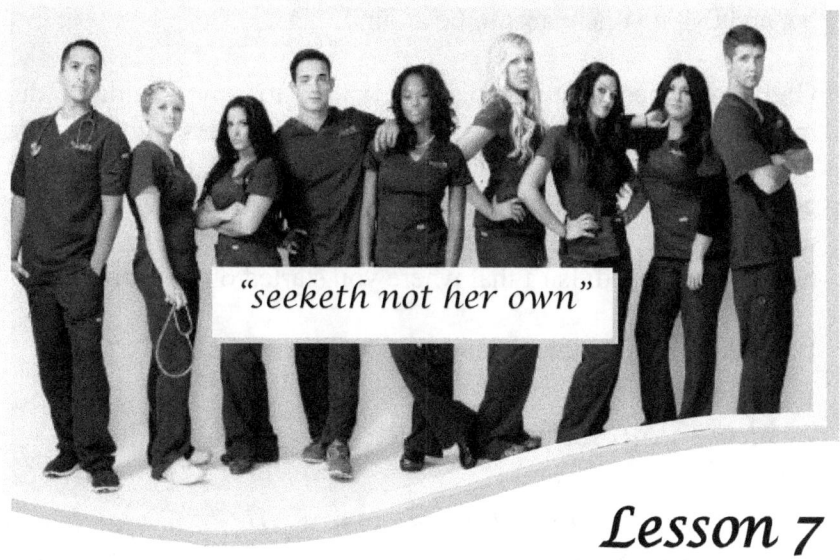

"seeketh not her own"

Lesson 7

When we were in high school, there were always those close-knit groups that roamed the halls acting snobbish to the rest of us. We called them "cliques" and in order to combat that, we formed our own "anti-clique cliques." In reality, most of our social structure is made up of these smaller "cliques" banded together by common interests and common backgrounds. Sometimes, even religion and race plays a part in whom we "hang out with." I'm sorry to say that high school was not the **last** place that you will find these groups.

Sometimes groups can be helpful, because it is there you find understanding of what you are dealing with. For example, other nurses on your floor see the same things you do, experience the same emotions you do, and may be frustrated with the same "red tape" that you are.

It's easy to fall back into the comfort and safety of their friendship. However, to build a wall around you and yours, may cause you to loose your willingness to venture out and be where you are actually needed. You will lose your edge if you are not careful, and will become the cynical, crabby, person that no one wants to be, and that no one wants to be around.

God challenges us, with this core value, to stay outside of our box. We are not to seek our own, but to seek others whom we can help. We must determine in our mind and heart that we are not going to be the person that needs to be propped up by others like us, but, rather, we will be the ones who step out of the crowd to help those in need. Isn't that where you started on this journey?

Here are some tips for maintaining that focus:

I. Make yourself a servant.

> *"For though I be free from all men, yet have I made myself servant unto all, that I might gain the more." 1Cor. 9:19*

Determine to be a servant. Yes, you know more about the medical field than the one for whom you are caring. Yes, you have much experience. Yes, you work closer to the patient and the patient's family than the doctor does, so you may be privileged to see things the doctor does not see. You will be tempted to seek out those who "see it your way," resulting in a group of followers. Suddenly, the work place, which has produced so much good, will become a toxic environment with everyone choosing sides as to who is right and who is wrong. Don't let that happen. Just do what you are supposed to do. Keep being a servant; let someone else be the boss.

II. Respect everyone.

> *"And unto the Jews I became as a Jew, that I might gain the Jews; to them that are under the law, as under the law, that I might gain them that are under the law; To them that are without law, as without law, (being not*

without law to God, but under the law to Christ,) that I might gain them that are without law. To the weak became I as weak, that I might gain the weak: I am made all things to all men, that I might by all means save some." 1Cor. 9:20-22

There is a lot of talk these days about tolerance for other religions and other political views. This is not a new concept. As a Christian, we are given the specific directive to be kind to those who differ from us.

God was very specific in the Old Testament that the Hebrew people were not to worship any other gods; in fact, many times they were told to destroy them. However, did you know that they were also specifically told not to "revile the gods"? (Ex. 22:28) The Lord said that He was a gracious God and, therefore, they were not to disrespect other's gods.

It is a good thing to let others know that you are interested in them. If they have some differences of opinion, let them express them. Then, be kind, listen and ask questions if you can, so that they feel that you are really listening to them.

III. Be sure of who you are.

"I therefore so run, not as uncertainly; so fight I, not as one that beateth the air:"
1Cor. 9:26

You are who you are. You believe what you believe. That's what makes you a unique person and a contributor to this life in which we are living. Don't forget who you are, and what you believe.

You can be sure that you are right, and still be kind. Sometimes, helping people that have a different world view than you have, can be difficult. Maybe, you are scandalized by the kind of life they live. Maybe their religion is completely different than anything you have ever encountered, and you are struggling with the things that you are required to do to make them feel comfortable. Don't forget who you are, but remember they are not you.

Several years ago I was called upon as a chaplain to help the families of some folks who had been involved in a shooting at a factory. All of the families were told to go to the local high school and wait to get news of their loved ones. The police had surrounded the factory and no one knew if the shooter was still alive, or if he had actually shot and killed anyone. The families were understandably distraught.

Many of them were smokers and were having trouble controlling their emotions. Normally, they would cope with the stress by lighting up a cigarette, but they couldn't because they were on school property. I am categorically against smoking, but was trying to understand their dilemma. We approached the school officials and created a smoking area for them. This diffused a situation that was becoming increasingly difficult to control. I did not begin to support smoking on school grounds, but that was not the time nor place to address this problem. Not everything you face will have a solution this simple, but I hope this illustrates how to implement this point.

IV. Be friendly to everyone.

> "And as ye would that men should do to you, do ye also to them likewise. For if ye love them which love you, what thank have ye? for sinners also love those that love them. And if ye do good to them which do good to you, what thank have ye? for sinners also do even the same." Luke 6:31-33

Have you ever thought about all the different kinds of people it takes to run a hospital or a nursing home? In the 1900's, a lady by the name of Isabel Briggs Myers, identified sixteen different personality traits that are used by most psychologists today. Her work was built on the work of another man named Carl Jung, and was first tested in the mid1900's on over 5,000 students.

After 30 years of research and thousands of people providing input—including her mother—her ideas were developed into a system of personality identification referred to as MBTI. (Myers-Briggs Type Indicator) A test was developed to determine the different personality types using four different preferences:

- **Extraversion or Introversion:** refers to where and how one directs his or her attention and energy on people and things in the outer world, or alone in the inner world.
- **Sensing or Intuition:** refers to how one prefers to deal with information by focusing on the basic information, or by interpreting and adding meaning.
- **Thinking or Feeling:** refers to decision making objectively, using logic and consistency, or subjectively, considering other people and special circumstances.
- **Judging or Perceiving:** refers to how one interacts with the outer world with a preference towards getting things decided, or for staying open to new information and options.

While it is true that everyone is an individual, and we should not stereotype and categorize people, it is also true that certain personality types are adept at certain things. There are different types of administrators and different kinds of administrations. Of course, fitting the right kind of administrator to the right kind of administration will produce the best results in any organization. But that is not what we are dealing with here.

Personalities have been narrowed down to four different types with each of these types having four subcategories:

Analysts

- ◆ **INTJ**—Imaginative and strategic thinkers, with a plan for everything.
- ◆ **INTP**—Innovative inventors with an unquenchable thirst for knowledge.
- ◆ **ENTJ**—Bold, imaginative and strong-willed leaders, always finding a way or making one.
- ◆ **ENTP**—Smart and curious thinkers who cannot resist an intellectual challenge.

Diplomats

- ◆ **INFJ**—Quiet and mystical, yet very inspiring and tireless idealists.
- ◆ **INFP**—Poetic, kind and altruistic people, always eager to help a good cause.
- ◆ **ENFJ**—Charismatic and inspiring leaders, able to mesmerize their listeners.
- ◆ **ENFP**—Enthusiastic, creative and sociable free spirits, who can always find a reason to smile.

Sentinels

- ◆ **ISTJ**—Practical and fact-minded individuals, whose reliability cannot be doubted.
- ◆ **ISFJ**—Very dedicated and warm protectors, always ready to defend their loved ones.
- ◆ **ESTJ**—Excellent administrators, unsurpassed at managing things, or people
- ◆ **ESFJ**—Extraordinarily caring, social and popular people, always eager to help.

Explorers

- ◆ **ISTP**—Bold and practical experimenters, masters of all kinds of tools.
- ◆ **ISFP**—Flexible and charming artists, always ready to explore and experience something new.
- ◆ **ESTP**—Smart, energetic and very perceptive people, who truly enjoy living on the edge.
- ◆ **ESFP**—Spontaneous, energetic and enthusiastic entertain-

ers—life is never boring around them.

You can find out more about these personality types, and even get a free analysis of your own personality type online. What I'd like you to think about in this context is that sometimes conflicts arise because people are different. Our world views are different. How we process things is different. Our backgrounds and experiences are different. To avoid the conflicts that inevitably arise, some of us will pull back into our little circles of friends and find comfort in criticizing those who are not like us. This is neither helpful nor healthy. It creates toxic work environments where people begin to hate their jobs and co-workers.

V. Stop looking for your soul mate.

There are love connection businesses that are built on trying to find a soul mate for you. The idea is, that if you can find a person that matches you—they like the same things that you like, etc.— then you can find a match that will last a life time. There are a few problems with that theory—the biggest one being that over time everyone changes. Appetites change. Abilities change. Associations change. Putting that aside, however, the biggest problem I see in this philosophy, is that people are basing their relationship on a completely selfish motive. They want to find someone that will be exactly like them.

When Jesus was asked the question, "Who is my neighbor?" He told of three people and their different reactions to a person who had been critically injured and left beside the road. You might remember this as the story of "The Good Samaritan," who took care of a wounded man whom he did not even know. The other men in the story passed by without helping. Jesus then completely flipped the question from "Who is my neighbor?" to "To whom are you a neighbor?"

We are not supposed to be looking to be a blessing to people like us. We are not supposed to stay in our comfort zones. We are supposed to reach out to those completely out of our racial, religious, and even personality circles, and show them kindness.

Reflection

What kind of personality do I have?
What weakness do I have in this area?

"Have patience. Remember how you will want someone to treat you when you reach the time when you need a caregiver!"

Linda D

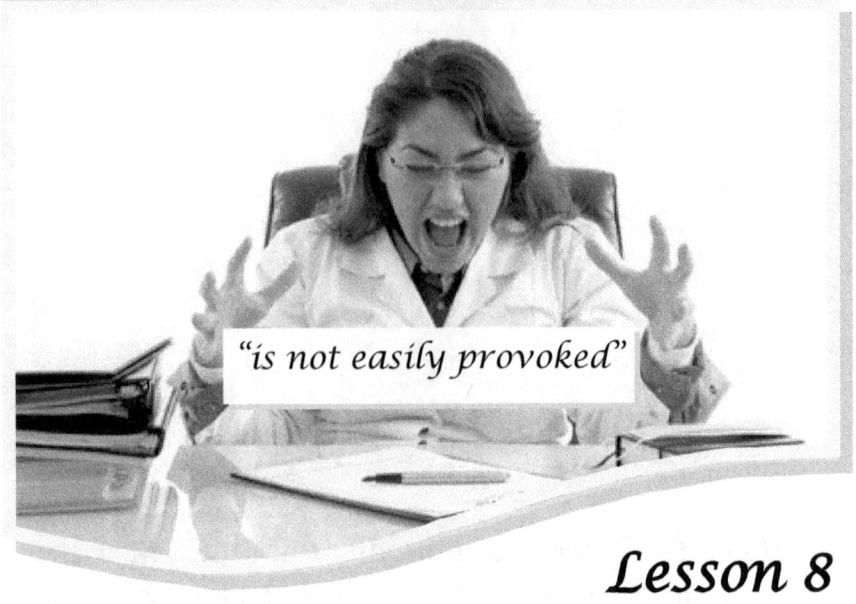

"is not easily provoked"

Lesson 8

Some people are easy to deal with and some are not. Some days you can deal with certain issues better than other days. What is important to remember is that you are a professional. You don't really have the luxury of reacting in a negative way to someone who is being a jerk...nor do you have the luxury of behaving badly just because you are having a bad day.

When you lose control of yourself, you are giving control of the situation to someone else. You might get angry and stomp away, thinking that you have made your point, but, in reality, you just left all of the decision-making power in the hands of other people. You might blow up hoping that your anger will force your will on those you are confronting, but all you have done is to create an opportunity for them to talk behind your back. You no longer will have the opportunity to discuss differences and come to logical conclusions. The Bible says it this way:

> *"He that hath no rule over his own spirit is like a city that is broken down, and without*

walls." *Pro. 25:28*

If you cannot control your spirit, someone else will control your life. Action builds things. Reaction destroys them. So how do you control your emotions? What can you do to keep the walls up around your personal city?

Your defenses must be built **before** the crisis not **during** the crisis. You must spend time working on who you are and developing your strength in peace time, so that you will be ready when the crisis comes. Here are some simple things to work on.

I. Build your confidence.

There is a verse in the Bible that goes like this:

> *"Great peace have they which love thy law: and nothing shall offend them."* *Psa. 119:165*

This verse simply means that if you love God's word, you will have great peace in your heart, and no one will be able to cause you to stumble. Several times throughout the Bible this same truth is echoed. Peace and confidence come from knowing that you are right with your relationship with God. It comes from placing your faith in what He has said and obeying His Word.

People can blow up around you. Circumstances can get difficult. But none of those things will even bother you, if your priorities are straight. If you know that you are doing right according to God's Word, and you trust God with all the details you will be completely unfazed by the contention of others.

II Humble yourself.

> *"Only by pride cometh contention: but with the well advised is wisdom."* *Pro. 13:10*

The only reason for a fight is pride. Two people disagree about something, and both of them want their way in the situation. I know that is not easy to accept, but it is true. A soft answer will always turn away wrath, but a soft answer will not come from the mouth of pride. An apology can fix a lot of hurts, but an apology will not come from a heart filled with pride.

Humility is not so much a state of mind as it is an action. The act of "humility" is not something you try to **be**. It is something you try to **do**. One of the challenges the Apostle Paul gives to those of the Philippian church is to esteem others better than themselves. This is difficult but necessary in the effort to be humble. Our natural inclination is to promote ourselves and our own ideas. We must—on purpose—decide to lift up other people and promote them and their ideas. Maybe your idea **is** better. If it is, it will come to the top. Meanwhile, be open to all other suggestions and ideas. Value all input as being more important than yours.

III. Think first—then speak.

> *"Even a fool, when he holdeth his peace, is counted wise: and he that shutteth his lips is esteemed a man of understanding."*
>
> Pro. 17:28

> *"Seest thou a man that is hasty in his words? there is more hope of a fool than of him."*
>
> Pro. 29:20

Words are a gift from God. In the very beginning, God created the heavens and the earth—with words. Words separate us from the animal kingdom. We communicate, encourage, network and build things with words.

However, words can also destroy. Just because you feel it—or think it—does not mean you should say it. You, and only you, have control of what comes out of your mouth.

Think on who is hearing what you are saying, not just on what you are saying. I've often heard someone say in anger, "I don't care who hears me say this..." The problem is that everyone that hears you can—and will—be affected in a different way. Maybe what is in your heart needs to be expressed, but in a controlled environment with the proper person to hear.

The Bible says that if you have something against a brother, you should first go to him privately, so that the difference can remain private. If you spread your anger around, other people will be infected with the "virus." You might even need to see a trusted counselor. who can hear your perspectives objectively. One who can help you craft a proper response and help you process the things you are thinking and feeling.

IV. Free up the clutter.

When someone loses his temper, it usually manifests a symptom of something that runs a lot deeper. Maybe there is a traumatic event in his past that has not been properly dealt with. Maybe he has experienced a great disappointment. Possibly he is overloaded with too many responsibilities. It's important to keep your life free of this kind of clutter.

If you have experienced a trying, traumatic experience, deal with it immediately. Most things get buried deep after 72 hours and will build up in the back of your mind and heart.

Sometimes in the middle of doing your job you don't think about the long-term affects it will have on you. It may not be until later, when you bite back at someone about nothing that you wonder, "Why did I respond that way?" It could be that you have been traumatized in a way that you don't realize. That doesn't mean you're crazy, nor does it mean that you need extended sessions with a "shrink." However, immediate intervention will most likely be all that is necessary to keep you balanced emotionally and professionally. Immediate intervention would include contacting your supervisor, and asking him to set up a "debriefing session" with a qualified specialist. That specialist can help you process what you have gone through, and possibly give you the tools to keep yourself spiritually and emotionally healthy.

Reflection

What can I do better to build myself spiritually?
Whom do I need to improve my attitude towards?
Do I typically react first and think later?
List some of the traumatic events that you have experienced which you have not talked to anyone about:

*"If you can't change your fate,
change your attitude."*

Amy Tan

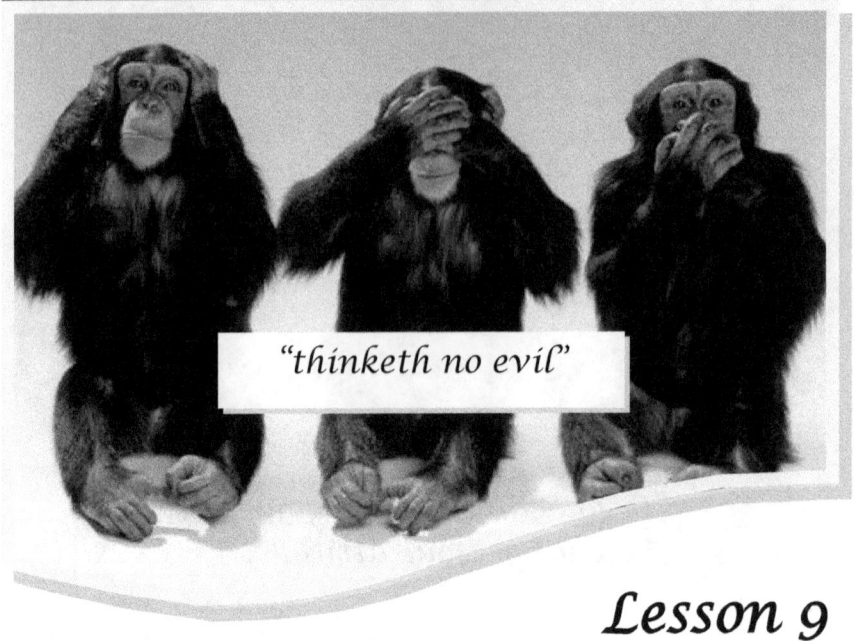

"thinketh no evil"

Lesson 9

At first glance, this statement, "thinketh no evil," appears to be a ridiculous requirement. No one can ignore the fact that evil is all around us. In fact, the older you get, the more prevalent it seems to be. Is God telling us to just pretend that there is no evil, and to go about our business without facing the realities around us? Of course not! Emphatically, NO! We are told over and over again that truth is critical for an effective Christian life. God never tells us to ignore or deny the truth. This phrase cannot possibly mean that. So what does it mean?

I. Do not think evil towards anyone.

Think for a minute about the core value we are studying, **Charity**. It has often been called, **Love in action**, because that is exactly what it is. A person with charity towards others, is one who doesn't wish evil on anyone.

The Bible is clear that we should not laugh at other's difficulties. It also instructs us to be very quick to forgive. These things go against our natural inclinations. We are quick to be snobbish and laugh at the idiosyncrasies of others. We are also quick to be involved in the "I told you so" moments, and the "I knew that was going to happen" gossip sessions. If someone does something against us, our natural desire is for vengeance or for them to get what's coming to them in return.

How much better it is to wish no evil on anyone. Hell is a place that even God, in all of His Holiness, doesn't want for us. That is why Jesus paid such a dear price to secure a place in heaven for us. Before we even knew there was a God, He made a way for us to be saved (Romans 5). God's thoughts about us are all good. He doesn't wish evil on anyone, and He expects us to behave in the same way.

II. *Keep evil thoughts from consuming you.*

Thinking is one of the greatest tools that God gave to us as humans, that He didn't give to the animal kingdom. Thinking allows us to come to conclusions through honest and viable thought processes—which all lead back to God, our Creator.

Imagination, on the other hand, can be our greatest nemesis. When God sent the flood to the earth, it was because of the wicked imaginations of man's heart (Genesis 6:5-13). Every thought man had just seemed to be bent towards evil. The problem is that every thought is simply the parent of the act. So evil thoughts will produce evil acts.

When Jesus came to earth, He shook up the religious world. Everyone was content to have a form of religion and to appear righteous, but was unwilling to deal with the heart issue. Jesus challenged the thinking more than the actions. The Apostle Paul echoes this same concept in his second letter to the Corinthians.

> *"Casting down imaginations, and every high thing that exalteth itself against the*

knowledge of God, and bringing into captivity every thought to the obedience of Christ."

1Cor. 10:5

This is what we are to be doing. We need to be constantly working at bringing our thoughts into obedience to Christ. We need to be casting down our evil imaginations.

III. Maintain a clean conscience.

"Unto the pure all things are pure: but unto them that are defiled and unbelieving is nothing pure; but even their mind and conscience is defiled." Titus 1:15

When you walk through the mud, you get mud on your shoes. Then everything that you walk on gets muddy, until all of the mud has been wiped off of your shoes. So it is with a dirty mind. If your thoughts are not clean, then everything you do will have the marks of sin on it. John tells us in his epistle (I John 1:9) that if we confess our sins to Christ, He will forgive us and cleanse us completely. Don't let the bad things stack up in your heart. As soon as you realize that you have thought wrong or done wrong, confess it to God and ask His forgiveness. He will immediately cleanse you, according to His Word.

Reflection

Do I think evil towards anyone?
What have I imagined that wasn't true?
What can I do to keep a clean conscience?

"*A merry heart doeth good like a medicine..*"

Proverbs 17:22

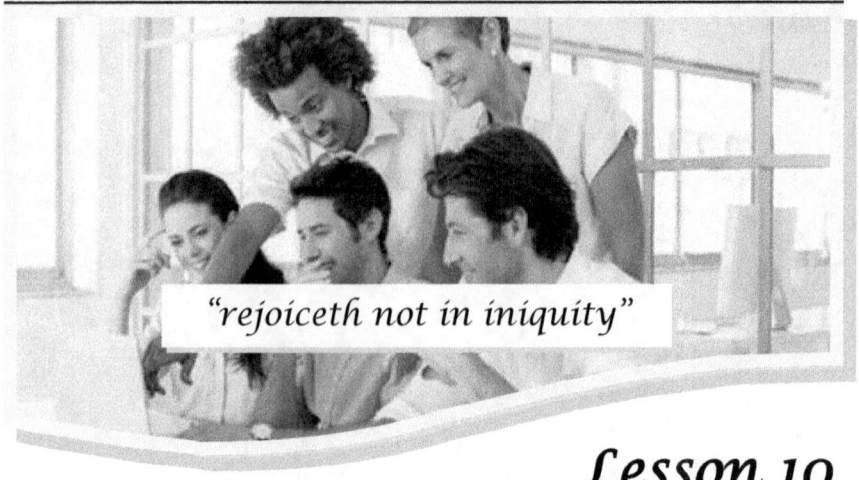

"rejoiceth not in iniquity"

Lesson 10

It is a common understanding that comedy influences the culture. While they may not specifically be setting out with that ideology in mind, comedians understand that people can take uncomfortable statements in a comical setting. Contemporary comedians consistently push the limits in racial issues, in sexual relationships, and even in areas like death and disease. Their main purpose is to get a laugh, but the natural conclusion of comedy is a shift in thinking. What was once taboo, becomes laughable and, in turn, acceptable.

The Bible warns us to stay away from "foolish jesting" and to not speak of those things that are "done of them in secret." I wonder if this is because what we laugh at is what shapes us. The Bible tells us that a "merry heart" is just like medicine. What if the medicine we take is the wrong prescription?

Here are some further thoughts to ponder on this subject:

I. Negative behavior produces negative results.

There is nothing positive about destructive behavior. It is not something we should laugh at, nor is it something we should hold in high esteem. What someone sows, they will reap. If you sow seeds of kindness, you will reap kindness from those around you. However, if you sow seeds of bitterness, you will reap bitterness. Don't make a mistake about sin or evil of any kind. Being party to it and rejoicing in it **will** produce regretful consequences.

II. Secretly enjoying evil produces a corrupt core.

In Romans chapter one. Paul describes the human condition without God. He goes into detail about sin and the places that the paths of sin leads us into. After explaining the condemnation on us because of the sin, he makes a profoundly strong statement:

"Who knowing the judgment of God, that they which commit such things are worthy of death, not only do the same, but have pleasure in them that do them." (Romans 1:32) In other words, if you enjoy watching someone else commit the sin, you are as guilty as they are. In another place Paul tells Timothy, "...neither be partaker of other men's sins." (I Timothy 5:22)

Not only are you guilty before God, but you have also brought their darkness into your own heart. We, as Christians, have the responsibility of bringing the light of Christ to this dark world. The more light there is, the more people can see the truth about themselves, their purpose, and their future.

We are supposed to be showing them the way back to their Creator, but when we partake of other men's sins, we have allowed the light that is in us to become darkness, and how great that darkness is! (Matthew 6:23) Our light, the potential for saving the lives and souls of other people, becomes dark, and then who will light the path to God? Who will light the path to hope?

As the rottenness inside of us grows, we will become more of a problem than a solution, and then when the storms of life blow through our lives, we will be nothing more than an empty tree, hollowed out by corruption.

III. Laughing at other people's calamity displeases God.

> *"Rejoice not when thine enemy falleth, and let not thine heart be glad when he stumbleth: Lest the LORD see it, and it displease him, and he turn away his wrath from him."*
> *Pro 24:17 -18*

A heart that is full of charity will not be glad when bad things happen to others. Don't be the kind of person who is always looking for someone to suffer the consequences of their actions. As a healthcare provider, you will often see people who are in bad physical condition as a result of their poor choices. If you choose to laugh at them, how can you help them?

Reflection

What am I tempted to laugh at that is wrong?
What can I do to keep from laughing at the calamities I see?

The truth is incontrovertible.
Malice may attack it, ignorance may deride it,
but in the end, there it is.

Winston Churchill

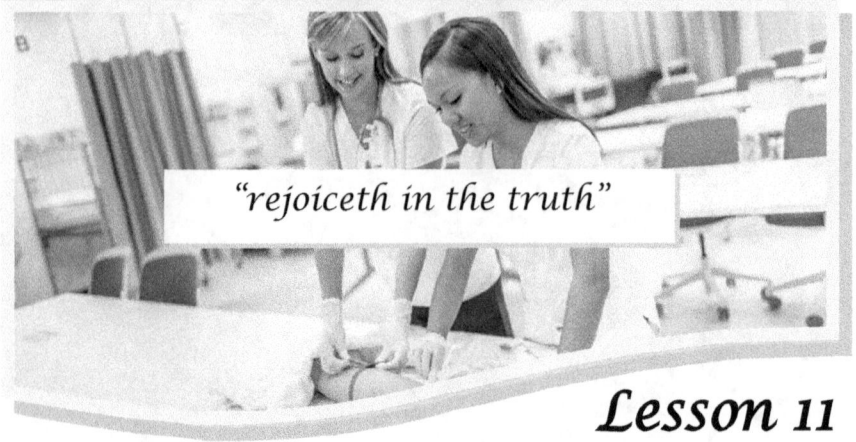

"*rejoiceth in the truth*"

Lesson 11

As Jesus stood before Pilate to be tried, Pilate asked Him if He were a king. Jesus' answer was that He had come to bear witness to the truth—to which the hardened Roman politician replied, "What is truth?"

Truth is what Jesus was all about. He was not trying to form a new religion using slick talk and illusions. He consistently brought people to reality. He seemed to have a specific interest in tearing down false religion, empty faith, and legalistic rules. His goal seemed to be to get to the heart of a person and change that heart.

Faith is often misunderstood. Faith in Christ is not to believe in the intangible. It is, instead, the complete embracing of truth in our lives. It is examining all of the evidence and coming to a logical conclusion. "Faith is the substance of things hoped for, the evidence of things not seen." (Hebrews 11:1)

As a Christian, truth should be the rule of our lives. Here are some things that the Bible teaches us about truth.

I. Truth is what sets us free.

> "*And ye shall know the truth, and the truth shall make you free.*" John 8:32

Telling lies to ourselves and others is a constricting activity. We have to remember what we said so that our story doesn't change. If we are living a life of lies, then we are constantly covering up—always afraid that someone will find out who we really are. Being completely honest with ourselves and others brings relief like nothing else. It takes away the need to appear to be something we are not.

Politicians are known for not keeping their promises, but every once in a while you find one with his integrity intact. One such politician told me that it is not hard being an honest politician if you remember two things. First, don't over commit yourself, and second, do what you say you are going to do. I think those are good rules to apply to anyone's life.

Paul tells us in II Timothy 2:25, that repentance—that is the turn around in our lives—is based upon our acknowledging of the truth. The Bible is a mirror that reflects our hearts. We are challenged to look into this mirror (James 1:2-26) and remember what we see. What we will see is not necessarily what we would like to see. However, an honest appraisal is the only thing that will help us make the changes that are necessary in our lives.

II. Truth is a behavior.

> *"But he that doeth truth cometh to the light, that his deeds may be made manifest, that they are wrought in God." John 3:21*

Truth is not just what you see and what you say; it is also a life style. Jesus said that doing truth has a way of guiding our steps closer to the light. More light exposes the flaws that we have, but it also shows us more of what God has done for us.

Lee Strobel is a journalist who was once an atheist. In his book, The Case for Faith, he describes his journey toward the light. His journey included the same questions many have asked like: "If there is a God, why is there so much suffering in the world?" There are many questions like this that beg to be answered by thinking people. The interesting thing is, that as you get closer and closer to truth, those questions have a way of making more sense. Doing truth is the decision to act only truthful in every way possible.

For example, in the book In His Steps, Charles Sheldon makes the point that most Christians talk about living a Christian life, but are not so willing to become what it really means to be a Christian. Christian is a term which means "Little Christ." It was a name given to the early believers as a term of derision. They called them such because all of those early believers were acting and talking like Christ. They said, "You are all just imitating Him." Of course, the church began to use the name as a badge of honor. Over time, it has lost its meaning. If a person believes that Jesus died on the cross he call himself a Christian—not because of what he does, but because of what he believes.

In Charles Sheldon's story, a preacher in a high society church makes a challenge to his people that for one year they follow the motto. "What would Jesus do?" in everything they did. The result of the experiment was a complete change in the town. The land-lords took better care of their tenants. The news media became more honest. The poor were taken care of, etc. This is a perfect example of what it means to do truth. Become what you say you are.

III. Faith can only grow in truth.

> "God is a Spirit: and they that worship him must worship him in spirit and in truth."
> John 4:24

Jesus did not leave any room to "fake it until we make it." He said in very clear terms that the only way to God was through Him. He said, "I am the way, the truth, and the life…" If you want a closer walk with God, then you cannot possibly live a life that is constantly manipulating and adjusting the truth.

We like to deal in perceptions. We want people to think highly of us, so we do things to cause them to perceive us as good. God doesn't work that way. He starts with where you really are, and then changes you into what you should be. He does not just treat symptoms. He gets to the root cause.

The good news is that you can be completely honest with Him. You don't have to pretend. You don't have to get your act together. You simply come to Him just as you are.

IV. Truth is the belt that binds our armor together.

> *"Stand therefore, having your loins girt about with truth, and having on the breastplate of righteousness." Eph. 6:14*

The Apostle Paul's letter to the Ephesians presents the struggles that we face in life as a battle—but not against people—against spiritual forces that are against us. He uses the armor of the Grecian soldier as an outline to help us understand how to defend ourselves and win against this darkness that is sometimes illusive.

Of course, He mentions the helmet and the breastplate. The helmet represents our own personal salvation. The breastplate is righteousness that protects us against the evil that would destroy our hearts.

The girdle of the Grecian soldier was often an ornamental piece which a soldier wore proudly. It was not just for decoration however, for it held a very important place in the armor of the soldier. First, it held the breastplate up tight against his chest, to both keep it in place—protecting the vital areas of the body—and also, to keep it from hindering the free movement of his body in a fight.

These are interesting comparisons to the value of truth in our lives. Honoring truth and keeping it as a major rule in our lives protects our heart from the evil around us. A life of truth also brings great confidence and freedom of movement to do what we are supposed to be doing.

Another use of the girdle was to hold the self defense weapons that were used up close. Daggers, short swords, and such were often kept in it. If a soldier found himself without any other weapon, his girdle would always have his back-up weapons much in the same way that the belts (of our modern soldiers) hold bullets and combat knives. So truth is always the back-up plan. You can be confident in it.

Yet one more use of the girdle was to hold a little bag called a scrip. The little bag might be comparable to a wallet or purse of today. In it, a soldier might have some dried meat and possibly a few coins to help him survive, wherever he might find himself. Once again can you see the value of truth? If you spend your life pulled together with truth, those things that are most personal and valuable to you will be kept safe.

Reflection

What people in my life do I need to be truthful with?
What do I need to be truthful about that will make a difference in my life?

"God gave burdens; He also gave shoulders."

Yiddish Proverb

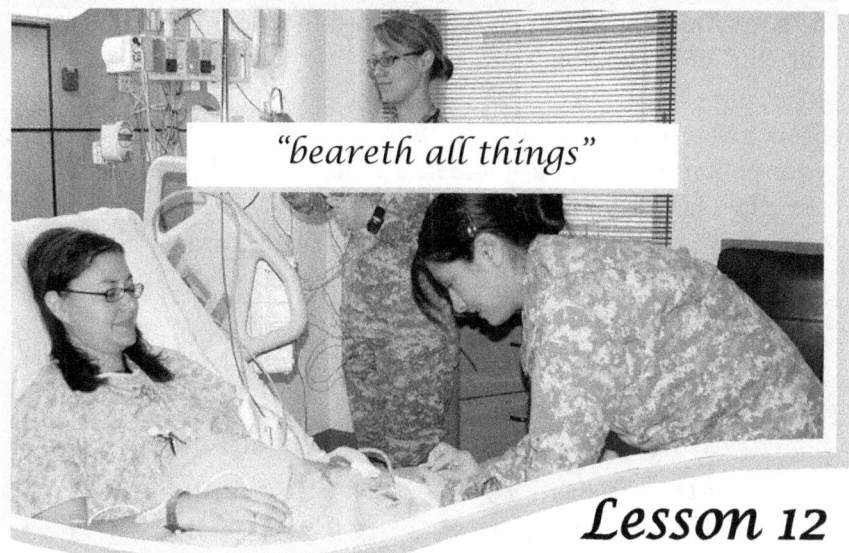

"*beareth all things*"

Lesson 12

Ok, how can you do this? Sometimes you might even get to the point where you have "caregiver's fatigue." That is, you come to where you just can't handle any more issues. How can you bear all things? Is it even possible to bear all the burdens that present themselves to you? Is that what this means?

Truly, everyone has his limit, but **you** are a caregiver. That is what your chosen profession is. How can you successfully and happily carry the burdens of others while you are juggling your own? That is what this lesson is about.

I. Genuinely care for your patient.

A story is told of a young orphan girl that took care of her little crippled brother in a country were children's services had not yet been developed. As the boy got older and consequently bigger, she found it increasingly difficult to pick him up and carry him as she had before. Someone happened by as she was trying to get him up off the ground onto her back to carry him to where they needed to go. That person, trying to help, kindly spoke up and said to her, "That is quite a burden you are carrying." The young girl, immediately, without hesitation, replied, "He's not a burden, he's my brother." Perspective helped this young lady deal with a very difficult situation.

Sometimes, because you deal with one case right after another, your patient becomes a number, a situation, and just a figure on the clipboard checklist. When that happens, you lose your ability to make the patient feel cared for. Don't stop caring. That is one of your most important jobs.

II. The yoke of Christ.

> *"Come unto me, all ye that labour and are heavy laden, and I will give you rest. Take my yoke upon you, and learn of me; for I am meek and lowly in heart: and ye shall find rest unto your souls. For my yoke is easy, and my burden is light." Mat. 11:28-30*

Farmers around the world have relied on well-trained oxen to plow their fields for generations. In some countries, it is still a common practice. Often a young ox will be placed in a double yoke with an older, seasoned ox to "learn" how to plow a straight furrow. Of course, the older—and usually stronger ox—will be the one pulling the weight. Sometimes it falls on him to pull the younger one along, as well as pull the load. This is the illustration that Jesus is giving to us. He obviously is the older and stronger ox, while we are the one that is still trying to figure out what in the world is happening to us.

When you develop a genuine relationship with Jesus Christ, you find a constant help in every struggle. You will find Him right there beside you, hearing every prayer, seeing every tear. Truthfully, He will carry the burden for you if you yield to His direction. Isaiah says, "But they that wait upon the LORD shall renew their strength; they shall mount up with wings as eagles; they shall run, and not be weary; and they shall walk, and not faint." (Is. 40:31)

III. Bear the burdens of one other.

Emergency response teams often have access to debriefing help after they have experienced a critical incident that was particularly traumatic. The International Critical Incident Stress Foundation (ICISF) was established to assist these caregivers in their own time of need and to equip specialists who could lead debriefing sessions. The ICISF team developed a strategy for helping in these types of extreme situations. This strategy is called "Critical Incident Stress Management" (CISM). Many have found it to be a helpful tool in dealing with their own burdens and the burdens of those around them.

CISM meets our basic need for someone to understand what we are going through, and it follows a detailed plan to help caregivers within seventy-two hours of a critical trauma.

The basic idea of the program is to sit down with those who have experienced the trauma and work back through it with them this way:

1- FACTS   First, the session leader asks the caregiver to describe the events of the trauma. Detail is good. Try to remember what all happened. Sometimes the events happen so fast that a person doesn't even have time to process it all. That is why this is so important.

2- REACTION   The second phase specifically focuses on the caregivers' reactions to the trauma. What did they do. How did they respond. Usually this reminds them that their training kicked in. and they did exactly what they were supposed to do. It is specifically important when there has been a death, because the caregiver feels his inadequacies and is faced with things out of his control.

3- EMOTION   The third phase deals with feelings. How did you feel when you saw this happen? What came into your mind?

Usually it connects to a previous trauma that you have experienced—possibly the death of a close family member, or some other type of crisis that overwhelmed you. Being honest at this point is so important, and afterward will bring such relief.

4- RE-ENTRY This phase is where the session leader reminds everyone how normal the reactions and feelings are. At this point I, personally, will give out a chart of the numerous reactions that can be experienced as a result of trauma, and folks will identify with many of them. Some type of instruction on how to relax and re-focus on that which is important is pertinent. Maybe, you need to go out on that date with your spouse or special friend, sit across the table and look into her/his eyes for a while. Maybe you need to go on to your kid's baseball game and sit and watch the game. Do not use alcohol to deal with the situation. Alcohol only complicates your feelings.

There are other steps and plans that are more detailed, but I have found this particular method to be very helpful in giving those caregivers staying power.

You can use this style of help with your friends and co-workers, no matter what the trauma. They will feel like a weight has been lifted off their shoulders, and you will find a solid friend to help you when you are in need. By the way, if your supervisor requires you to go to a debriefing, don't disregard it. Participate and you will find soul-healing.

IV. Don't forget to take a vacation.

The best cure for stress is sleep. Don't cheat on your rest. Some folks require more sleep than others. Listen to your body and know when you need to stop and sleep.

There was a time when Jesus forced a vacation on the disciples. They had just come back from a mission outreach a distance away from Him, where they had been healing the sick and casting out demons on their own. When they came back to Him, they found out that John the Baptist had been brutally murdered and they were stunned. While they were trying to process their own personal elation and sudden grief, thousands of people began congregating around Jesus to hear Him teach. As His sermon lasted late into the day, the people began to be hungry. Jesus asked for the disciples to assist Him in setting the people down on the hillside. Jesus then took five loaves and two fishes, divided them up and sent the disciples out to give the food to everyone. When everyone had finished eating, they had to clean it all up and picked up twelve baskets full of leftovers and scraps. Now they were really tired. The Bible says that at this time Jesus constrained them to get on a boat and go away—not to go away permanently, but just to get away from the crowd for a little bit to rest and recuperate.

Vacation is important. It is not a badge of honor to work for many years without taking a break. That is insanity.

Reflection

What do you know about your current patients?
Describe your dream vacation:
What is the date of your next vacation?

"I believe in Christianity as I believe that the sun has risen: not only because I see it, but because by it I see everything else."

C.S. Lewis

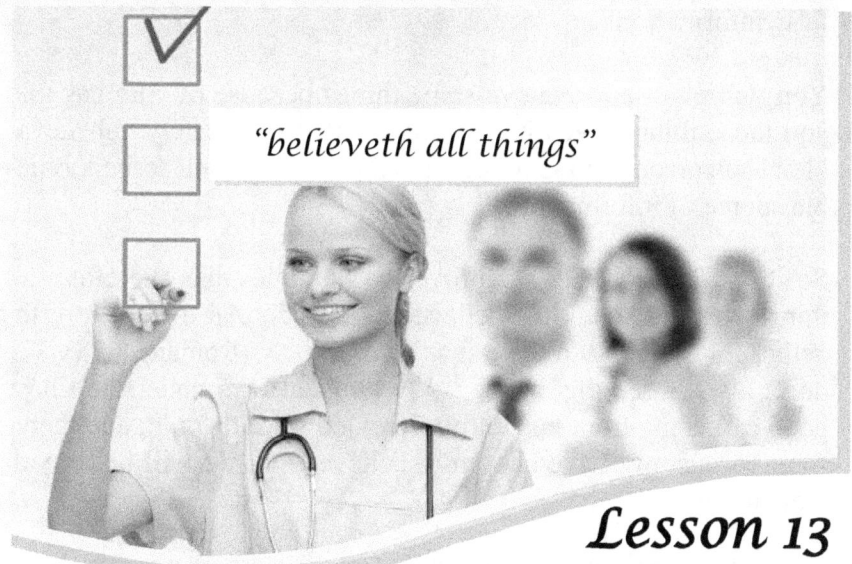

"believeth all things"

Lesson 13

You have probably heard the phrase, "There's a sucker born every minute." P.T. Barnum, founder of the Barnum and Bailey Circus, is credited for the saying. Interestingly enough, this statement was made by someone else about the crowds that Barnum would draw to see his famous hoaxes.

To believe everything you hear or see, is to be gullible and vulnerable. Current media outlets, both social and corporate, have aptly demonstrated how easily the truth can be manipulated. So must we be gullible to exhibit true charity? No.

Paul is not speaking generally here, that we should believe everything we hear. Instead, his point is one that is a reflection of all of the Bible. The fact is, that faith is believing all that God has said—even the parts we don't understand. Believing all things that God has told us is the source of life and happiness.

I. Belief is a choice.

You choose to believe things based on what you can accept as truth. Sometimes you might find yourself believing things that are not true, because you were merely basing your assumptions on false information.

You will choose to believe some things because of who has told you those things, even if the story itself is completely unbelievable. The person who is telling it has proven himself to be a reliable source of information.

So it is with God. He has proven to be believable, therefore, all things He says should be believed. He said, "All things work together for the good to them that love God…" (Romans 8:28). We don't always see this happen. We don't always understand how good can come from evil. However, God said it would, and therefore, because we have chosen to believe God, we will believe all that He says.

In the book <u>The Case for Faith</u> by Lee Strobel, the author recounts a discussion he had with a noted philosopher, Peter Kreeft, about why God allows suffering in the world. Kreeft explained to him that God in His infinite wisdom knows that short-term grief can mean long-term benefit. Stroble asked how this was possible, to which Kreeft replied, "…He has demonstrated how the very worst thing that has ever happened in the history of the world ended up resulting in the very best thing that has ever happened in the history of the world." He went on to explain that the death of Christ on the cross—literally the death of God—resulted in opening heaven to human beings. "So," he said, "the worst tragedy in history brought about the most glorious event in history." The ultimate evil resulted in the ultimate good.

So we can believe everything He says even when it doesn't make sense.

II. Everything that pertains to life is rooted in what you believe.

> *"According as his divine power hath given unto us all things that pertain unto life and*

godliness, through the knowledge of him that hath called us to glory and virtue." I Pet. 1:3

Everything you do in life is rooted in what you believe. If you believe **some** things that God says and yet you don't believe other things, then you will choose to live your life in a way that is convenient to you alone.

How you treat your patients is a direct reflection of whether or not you believe, as God said, that they were created in the image of God. So what, if they are being difficult today! That doesn't mean that they weren't created with a valuable purpose. So their bad choices have resulted in their bad health, they are still a valuable part of God's creation.

As you read through the Bible, one thing becomes abundantly clear: no one is perfect. Not one of us can even hope to come close to perfection. The best of the best in the Bible had critical flaws that would easily exclude them from living in the presence of God. Yet time and time again, God would forgive them.

The common denominator for all of those who were followers of God is that they all believed Him. Abraham believed God and that was counted unto righteousness (Romans 4:3).

The book of Colossians tells us that Jesus took all of the ordinances that were against us—that is, all of the ordinances that we could not possibly keep—and nailed them to His cross. He then established faith as the key to a righteous life. Faith is the source of goodness; faith is the source of permanent change.

III. What you believe, will affect your behavior.

"But without faith it is impossible to please him: for he that cometh to God must believe that he is, and that he is a rewarder of them that diligently seek him." Hebrews 11:6

The Bible has much to say about rewards. Over and over again, we are told that the Lord sees what we do in secret and will reward us openly. The desire for reward is a strong motivator. If you believe that the good that you do will be noticed and rewarded, you will be more prone to do good.

Consider these verses:

Mat. 6:6 "But thou, when thou prayest, enter into thy closet, and when thou hast shut thy door, pray to thy Father which is in secret; and thy Father which seeth in secret shall reward thee openly."

Mark 9:41 "For whosoever shall give you a cup of water to drink in my name, because ye belong to Christ, verily I say unto you, he shall not lose his reward."

Luke 6:35 "But love ye your enemies, and do good, and lend, hoping for nothing again; and your reward shall be great, and ye shall be the children of the Highest: for he is kind unto the unthankful and *to* the evil."

Col. 3:24 "Knowing that of the Lord ye shall receive the reward of the inheritance: for ye serve the Lord Christ."

Heb. 10:35 "Cast not away therefore your confidence, which hath great recompence of reward."

Heb. 11:26 "Esteeming the reproach of Christ greater riches than the treasures in Egypt: for he had respect unto the recompense of the reward."

2 Jn. 1:8 "Look to yourselves, that we lose not those things which we have wrought, but that we receive a full reward."

Rev. 11:18 "And the nations were angry, and thy wrath is come, and the time of the dead, that they should be judged, and that thou shouldest give reward unto thy servants the prophets, and to the saints, and them that fear thy name, small and great; and should-est destroy them which destroy the earth."

Rev. 22:12 "And, behold, I come quickly; and my reward *is* with me, to give every man according as his work shall be."

Because God is the One Who ultimately rewards us for our deeds, we are to behave as if He were our boss. Everything we do is to be done in a way that would please Him. This mentality will cause your work to be performed well, even when no one is inspecting you. Of course, others will notice the conscientious way in which you conduct yourself, and you will find the side benefits like Joseph did.

Reflection

What do I believe about God?

How has this belief affected my life?

Are there areas where I could be more conscientious?

"*Hope is the thing with feathers*
That perches in the soul
And sings the tune without the words
And never stops at all."

Emily Dickinson

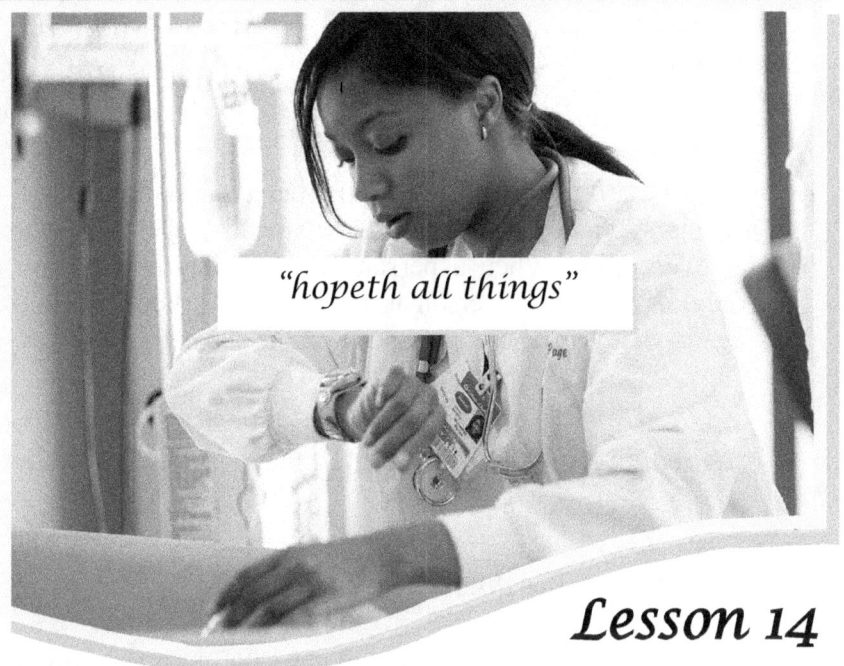

"hopeth all things"

Lesson 14

In the early 1900's, Thomas Edison said, "The doctor of the future will give no medicine, but will instruct his patient in the care of the human frame, in diet and in the cause and prevention of disease." His prediction has come true in the sense that many medical doctors and health facilities have taken what has become known as the "holistic" approach to medicine. If you are reading this as a health professional, you certainly have come across this term already.

The main idea of holistic medicine is to treat the whole person. Just medicine does not heal people. Meditation, spiritual guidance, and new life choices are being touted as fundamental to our well being. Long before Edison, a Jewish king named Solomon made similar claims:

> *"A merry heart doeth good like a medicine: but a broken spirit drieth the bones." Pro. 17:22*

"Hope deferred maketh the heart sick: but when the desire cometh, it is a tree of life."
Pro. 13:12

Hope makes a difference in healing. If a person has something to live for, his survival rate increases dramatically, even when his odds are very slim. When a person gives up, he quickly fails. Truthfully, as long as a person is alive, there is hope for him. Once again, wise King Solomon spoke on the subject:

"For to him that is joined to all the living there is hope: for a living dog is better than a dead lion." Ecc. 9:4

I. Hope will bring positive action.

Did you know that Thomas Edison made 1,000 unsuccessful attempts at making the light bulb. When a reporter asked, "How did it feel to fail 1,000 times?" He replied, "I didn't fail 1,000 times. The light bulb was an invention with 1,000 steps."

There are countless stories like this of successful men and women. The common denominator in all of their success stories is that they refused to give up. Hope drove them to succeed.

When Abraham was nearly 100 years old, God promised him that he would have a son. Because the possibility of a man at that age producing a child is pretty much miraculous, the Bible says this on the subject:

"Who against hope believed in hope, that he might become the father of many nations, according to that which was spoken, So shall thy seed be." Rom. 4:18

Hope will cause you to act in a certain way, and a lack of hope will cause you to act exactly opposite. Hope produces. Hopelessness destroys.

II. *Hope will provide vision.*

> *"For we are saved by hope: but hope that is seen is not hope: for what a man seeth, why doth he yet hope for? But if we hope for that we see not, then do we with patience wait for it." Rom 8:24-25*

Hope will help you see a positive end to a difficult situation. It will help you have confidence when the storms of life are raging around you. Hopelessness will blind you to the possibilities.

III. *Hope will be an anchor.*

> *"Which hope we have as an anchor of the soul, both sure and stedfast, and which entereth into that within the veil." Heb. 6:19*

When things don't look right; when they don't make sense, hold on to the truth that there is a God in heaven who is watching and waiting for you to trust Him. Within the veil of the Jewish temple was the mercy seat where God met with man. It is there that we find confidence. He cares about us. He wants to be with us, and we can be sure of His presence in our lives.

Reflection

What will you choose to hope about?

"Be determined to handle any challenge in a way that will make you grow."

Les Brown

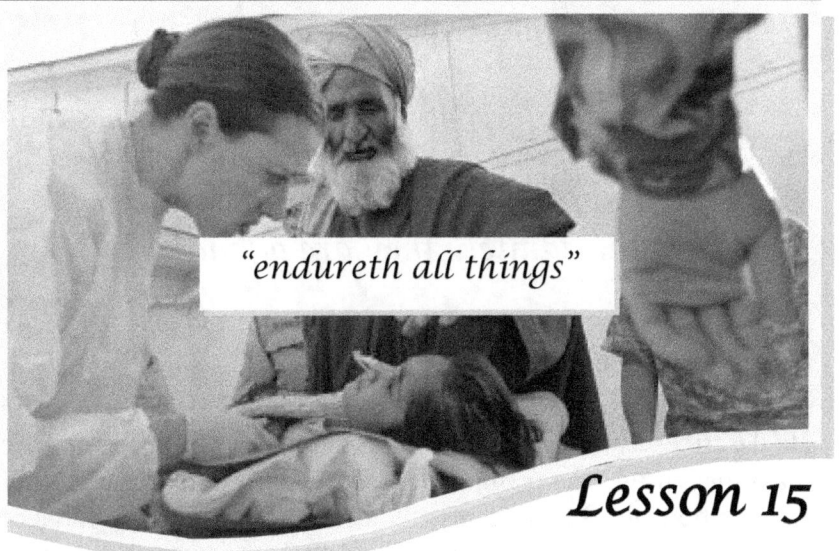

"endureth all things"

Lesson 15

Most stories of endurance are about fabulous athletic feats. For example, there is the man who swam the Atlantic Ocean, and the guy who ran five ironman triathlons in five days, and don't forget the guy who spent over an hour immersed in ice just to break his previous world record of the same nature.

One story that really caught my attention, however, is a little Indian man named Dashrath Manjhi. He was not a super athlete or daredevil. His wife died due to lack of medical treatment because the nearest doctor was 70 km away from his village. He did not want anyone else to suffer the same fate, so for 22 years he worked carving a cut through the mountain to form a road. His efforts reduced the travel distance from the Atri to Wazirganj areas of the Gaya district from 75km to 1km. I was impressed, not just with his endurance, but with the love and care for his wife and his people that motivated such extreme effort.

As a healthcare professional, you have a cause worth the effort. The things you must endure—although difficult—produce results that will long outlast your life; therefore, you must learn to endure.

I. Endurance comes from an internal root.

> *"And have no root in themselves, and so endure but for a time: afterward, when affliction or persecution ariseth for the word's sake, immediately they are offended."*
>
> Mark 4:17

In this passage, Jesus is teaching about the four different kinds of soil that receive the seed—The Word of God. This particular soil He describes as rocky and hard. The seed may germinate, and the plant may grow. The plant might even begin to show evidence of just a little fruit. But suddenly, the heat of the sun or the force of the wind destroys the plant completely. That is because there is no solid root.

It is just the same in the life of an individual. If there is no root down deep, no spiritual core, then difficulty will cause one to wilt and fall apart. The only way to be sure that you can handle the pressure that your job and life together throw at you, is to be sure that you are rooted deep in the promises of God and in a solid relationship with Him.

II. Endurance is hard.

> *"Thou therefore endure hardness, as a good soldier of Jesus Christ."* 2 Tim 2:3

Make no mistake about it, enduring is hard. Easy things are not **endured**. Fun things are not **endured**; only things that tax us beyond our limits are endured.

Whenever the subject of endurance comes up, we often hear the name Shackleton. He is mentioned because of the incredible experience that he and his crew had to endure while attempting to cross the Antarctic. The reason that this epic adventure became synonymous with endurance is not due to Shackleton and his leadership skills, however. It is because of an Australian photographer, named Frank Hurley. He was always scaling some dangerous precipice, climbing the icy mast, or some other crazy stunt just to get good pictures of the whole event. His legendary pictures have chronicled the events in such a way as to capture the imagination of all armchair explorers.

As the expedition dragged on, many of the crewmembers became discouraged and began to unravel emotionally. It is said that Hurley was amazed at their lack of fortitude and stamina. While they were cowering in shelters, bundled up to their eyeballs in coats and blankets, Frank Hurley (with the gusting, freezing wind disheveling the hair of his unprotected head) was out on the ice with his camera, moving this way and that in an attempt to capture the best angles—recording the event in pictures. It was his endurance, beyond the limits of the rest, that gave us a peek into one of the most amazing stories of survival ever to be told.

It would seem that the greatest endurance always yields the greatest rewards.

You are a soldier. You are on the front lines of battle. Your endurance will make a difference in the life of others. So, hold on. Be strong. Make a difference.

III. Endurance yields eternal rewards.

> *"For this is thankworthy, if a man for conscience toward God endure grief, suffering wrongfully. For what glory is it, if, when ye be buffeted for your faults, ye shall take it patiently? but if, when ye do well, and suffer for it, ye take it patiently, this is acceptable with God." 1Peter 2:20*

- *Core Centered Care* -

This verse states that endurance is "thankworthy." The word simply means "worthy of thanks." Worthy of thanks from whom? Who is going to thank us for enduring? God is the one doing the thanking!

Peter is describing the ultimate Christian response to adversity. We are to follow in the steps of Christ, who did not threaten when He could have. Instead, when He was suffering a wrongful death, He uttered words of forgiveness and hope to all those around Him. He tells John to take care of His mother. He tells the thief hanging beside Him that they will meet again that very day in Paradise. He tells the Father to forgive the blasphemy of the Pharisees, because they do not know what they are doing. All of these things He does for the very ones who put Him on the cross.

Don't pat yourself on the back for humbly accepting correction. No, Peter is not praising us for behaving in a proper manner. He is telling us to respond humbly and kindly when we are being chastised and criticized—even when we don't deserve it.

Oh, I understand how hard this is. Indeed, it is not possible without supernatural intervention. You cannot possibly act like Christ without His Spirit in you.

I find it interesting that God will say thank you to us for doing what He gives us the power to do. He is the one that fills us with love. He, alone, gives us the strength to forgive those who trespass against us. He went to the cross because of us. Yet, He will say, "Thank you," to us for acting like He did.

This is the attitude we are to have. Quiet forgiveness and help to those who are doing us wrong. This is what God says is acceptable.

IV. Endure to the end.

Sometimes after we have done all that God has asked of us, we become weary. The difficulty of trying to do right when no one else seems to care, soon becomes a heavy burden. We look around us and no one else is doing right, and so little by little we let down our guard. Step by little step we wander off the path that God has called us to, then one day we wake up to find ourselves a long way from where we once were.

Peter found himself in that same exact spot. However, what he discovered was that all the while he was walking away, Jesus was watching. When he found himself in a situation he could not extract himself from, he cried out to God. Quickly and lovingly the Great Physician healed his heart and restored him to spiritual health.

When you are enduring a trial, you may feel weak. That's ok. It's common. Don't be afraid to call for help. When you fall—and you might—just get back up again and keep going.

Reflection

What situation am I facing that I need to endure?
What things have I dropped that I need to get back to?